Essential Oils For Your Pet

47 Safe, Natural And Easy Home
Remedies For Fido
(Aromatherapy for Dogs)

CORAL MILLER

DEDICATION

To Rockie, Coco and Lexi, my furry companions, you make life fun!

TABLE OF CONTENT

INTRODUCTION

Essential Oils And Your Pet

People keep pets for different reasons: for companionship, for protection, for exercise and weight loss or for their looks or specific breed. Whatever valid reason it may be, all pets require effective healthcare and what better, safer, cheaper and all-natural way to go about this than to use essential oils and aromatherapy.

Essential oils are highly concentrated substances extracted from the leaves, bark, bushes, flowers, roots, fruits, shrubs or seeds of plants. They are responsible for providing plants with their powerfully unique scents, while enhancing their immune system and offering the necessary protection. They can be extracted in different ways such as steam distillation, carbon dioxide extraction, solvent extraction or manual expression. Each essential oil comes with its own individual scent, healing benefits, color and chemical properties.

As mentioned earlier, Essential oils are safer, cheaper, and more effective healthcare alternative for fido. Dogs respond very well to it once it is used appropriately. It can be used to treat numerous ailments ranging from allergies and its accompanying symptoms (itchy, dry, flaky skin),

skin infections and conditions (wounds, bumps, eczema,), arthritis / muscular issues, respiratory and digestive issues as well as emotional and behavioral concerns (stress, fear, anxiety).

However, for aromatherapy to effectively tackle dog health problems, certain factors must be considered. Topmost on the list is the purity of the essential oils utilized. Only the purest essential oils in the market must be used. The essentials oils must have a "Therapeutic Grade" rating. If you use aromatherapy grade or perfume quality oils for topical application, for example, you may be doing more harm than good because the oils are distilled using solvents. Pure therapeutic grade oils are steam distilled and do not contain any chemicals.

The price indicates its level of purity. Pure therapeutic essential oils are usually more costly. So if you see cheaper essential oils in the market, do not buy as they may be adulterated. The oils must also be bottled in cobalt, violet or amber glass bottles.

Another important factor is dilution and dosage. Dilution has to do with the amount of essential oils that is present in a blend while dosage is the amount of the blend that is administered to the dog such as drops.

Diluting Essential Oils For Dogs

Essential oils must be diluted according to the size of the dog. For small dogs that are between 5-15 pounds, essential oil dilution ratio is 90%. For Small-Medium dogs that are between16-30 pounds, the dilution ratio is 75%. Medium dogs, 31-50 pounds would have a 50% dilution of the essential oil.

s/n	Size of Dog	Weight (lb)	Essential Oil Dilution Ratio
1	small dogs	5- 15 lb	90%
2	small-medium dogs	16-30 lb	75%
3	medium dogs	31-50 lb	50%
4	large dogs	51-89lb	25%
5	extra large dogs	90lb and over	undiluted

The amount of dilution also depends on the type of essential oil. Lavender and roman chamomile oils for instance are gentle and so may not require much dilution. Lavender can even be used without dilution. Strong essential oils like oregano, clove and thyme must always be diluted accordingly.

The response should also be monitored. Response either positive or negative occurs immediately or several days later. If there is no response, try another essential oil. If there is a negative response such as mild pinkness of the skin or mild watering of the eyes, let your pet rest for 24-48 hours then try another essential oil.

This is another reason you should use 100% pure essential oils, it is safe for dogs and usually do not cause adverse effects. If using oil for the first time, introduce it to the dog in small amounts to see if it upsets him. He shows this by it by panting, drooling or whining. Start with gentle oil and then and work up to the stronger ones.

Always dilute with a pure carrier and not water. Also, correct adverse reaction with pure carrier oil by using to wash the affected area. For dosage, small dogs require fewer amounts of diluted oils while bigger dogs will need a larger amount.

Essential Oils Benefits for Dogs

1. It is non-toxic to the body. It is safe to apply and leave no side effects.

2. It is easy to use. Dogs can inhale essential oils directly from the bottle or from your hand. You can also apply directly on their paw or body.

3. Extremely versatile, essential oils address a wide range of issues such as motion sickness, tick removal and stomach problems. They are very effective as well.

4. They increase alertness for pets as they age. They help to reestablish old habits so the pets maintain their level of alertness even as they grow old. Cedarwood, frankincense, sandalwood, lavender, vetiver and lemon oils are examples.

5. They are great training aids for emotions. They can be used to calm anxiety and to make dogs concentrate.

6. They improve coat and skin. Essential oils help the skin to regenerate, its antioxidant effects helps to restore health to the coat.

7. They are safe cleaning agents. There is no fear of your pets ingesting caustic cleaners while drinking from toilet bowls or licking areas where such cleaners are used. Lemon, rosemary, and eucalyptus oils are examples.

8. Helps to eliminates odors. Use essential oils to eliminate pet odors and stains and keep your home smelling nice all day long.

Safe Essential Oils For Dogs

While essential oils provide a range of treatments for your pets, they are not all safe for your dogs. Below are a few popular oils that you can safely use on your dogs.

Lavender

A "must-have" for your dog, lavender oil is a good first aid that is extremely safe and gentle. It is antibacterial and helps to treat common animal ailments such as skin irritations and itches. It calms and soothes. It can be used diluted or undiluted.

Bergamot

Antifungal and soothing, this essential oil helps to fight ear infections caused by bacterial overgrowth or yeast. However, it can cause photosensitization so your pet must stay away from the sun after use.

Chamomile, Roman

It is analgesic and antispasmodic. It helps to soothe the central nervous system. It provides relief from cramps, muscle pains and teething pain. It is very important for dogs.

Helichrysum

Anti-inflammatory and analgesic oil, helichrysum is an excellent skin regenerator. It is great for skin conditions such as eczema. It reduces bleeding in accidents. It helps heal scars and bruises and it is effective for pain relief.

Niaouli

Although Niaouli has powerful antibacterial properties, it is gentle on the skin. It works wonderfully on ear infections and skin troubles caused by allergies.

Peppermint

Antispasmodic, peppermint stimulates circulation. It can be combined with ginger essential oil to effectively treat motion sickness. It also helps with arthritis, sprains and strains. Repel insects as well.

Geranium

Antifungal, it is gentle and safe, good fungal ear infections and skin irritations. It is an effective tick repellant.

Valerian

It helps to calm nerves and thus good for treating anxiety in dogs.

Eucalyptus Radiata

It is antiviral and anti-inflammatory. An effective expectorant, it provides relief from chest congestion. It also repels fleas.

German Chamomile

This oil works well on burns, stings and good for allergic reactions.

Essential Oil Precautions With Dogs

• Always dilute essential oils with a carrier oil like olive oil or coconut oil. To guide you, add about 10 to15 drops of essential oils to 15 ml (1/2 oz) of carrier oil.

• Use cautiously with pregnant dogs, puppies under 10 weeks of age or very old dogs. As a matter of fact, check with your vet before using on pregnant dogs.

• Avoid nose, eyes, anal, anal area and genital areas.

• Always use 100% therapeutic grade essential oils that is pure and non- adulterated.

• Do not use oils on seizure-prone or epileptic dogs.

• Do not try to treat seriously injured dogs. Consult your vet.

• Less is more! Being conservative with essential oil is safer than being liberal. Dogs' olfactory sensitivity is reported to be about 100 times greater than humans. They can detect odorant molecules at a really lower concentration.

• Do not use these oils on dogs: pennyroyal, wormwood, rue, horseradish, birch, wintergreen, camphor, clove leaf, cassia and anise.

• Always wash your hands after applying oils so it doesn't accidentally get into your eyes.

• Do not add your 100% pure essential oils to synthetic shampoos, laundry soaps, detergents. Use all natural bases instead.

How To Apply Essential Oils To Dogs

<u>Topically</u>

Topical application is the most common of all as it provides the greatest benefits. The oils are applied directly to the area (s) of concern and are quickly absorbed into the bloodstream. The ears, toes, pads and spine of dogs are common examples. Essential oils can also be applied directly to the wound or via massage. However, avoid getting it into the eyes, nose, anal and genital areas. The oils can be added to shampoos, ointments, conditioners, salves, etc as well.

<u>Aromatically</u>

Essential oils can be applied aromatically via inhalation and diffusion. You can put a drop of essential oil on his collar or on the dog bed. He can even inhale from your hands.

Spritzers or sprays can also be used by mixing essential oil and water and spraying on fur.

A diffuser helps to evaporate the oils which are then inhaled by the dog. For your pet to inhale and absorb the essential oils very well, leave the diffuser on for at least 30 minutes. You may do this procedure twice daily for a week so as to get positive result.

Internally

Never administer essential oils to your pets internally unless under supervision of a veterinarian. Remember they are highly concentrated and potent so take extreme care so you do not administer overdose. Even when you get a vet's approval, do not administer more than 1 drop in an empty capsule for your dog. The oils must also be Certified Pure Therapeutic Grade.

ESSENTIAL OIL DOG BATH RECIPES

Calming Shampoo
Make your dog relax after a bath

What You Need

2 drops vetiver essential oil

4 drops petitgrain essential oil

3 drops valerian essential oil

2 drops sweet orange essential oil

3 drops sweet marjoram essential oil

8 oz (240ml) all natural shampoo base

<u>Directions</u>

1. Add oils to shampoo.

2. Shake thoroughly and use.

Puppy Shampoo

<u>What You Need</u>

5 drops geranium essential oil

5 drops petitgrain essential oil

2 drops rose essential oil

2 drops ylang ylang essential oil

2 drops roman chamomile essential oil

8 oz (240ml) all natural shampoo base

<u>Directions</u>

1. Add oils to shampoo.

2. Shake thoroughly and use.

Tick Repelling Shampoo
<u>What You Need</u>

2 drops rosewood essential oil

3 drops lavender essential oil

2 drops geranium essential oil

2 drops myrrh essential oil

1 drops bay leaf essential oil

2 drops opoponax essential oil

8 oz (240ml) all natural shampoo base

<u>Directions</u>

1. Add oils to shampoo.

2. Shake thoroughly and use.

Flea/ Insect Repelling Shampoo
<u>What You Need</u>

2 drops citronella essential oil

4 drops clary sage essential oil

4 drops lemon essential oil

8 drops peppermint essential oil

8 oz (240ml) all natural shampoo base

Directions

1. Add oils to shampoo.

2. Shake thoroughly and use.

Spicy Deodorant Shampoo
What You Need

4 drops atlas cedarwood essential oil

2 drops patchouli essential oil

4 drops rosemary essential oil

 3 drops vetiver essential oil

8 oz (240ml) all natural shampoo base

Directions

1. Add oils to shampoo.

2. Shake thoroughly and use.

Delicate Floral
What You Need

6 drops petitgrain essential oil

4 drops lavender essential oil

4 drops rose essential oil

2 drops ylang ylang, essential oil

8 oz (240ml) all natural shampoo base

Directions

1. Add oils to shampoo.

2. Shake thoroughly and use.

Refreshing Citrus Shampoo
What You Need

3 drops grapefruit essential oil

3 drops lemon essential oil

3 drops lime essential oil

3 drops sweet orange essential oil

3 drops mandarin essential oil

8 oz (240ml) all natural shampoo base

Directions

1. Add oils to shampoo.

2. Shake thoroughly and use.

Fresh Herbal Shampoo

<u>What You Need</u>

4 drops clary sage essential oil

4 drops sweet basil essential oil

4 drops coriander seed essential oil

4 drops lavender essential oil

8 oz (240ml) all natural shampoo base

<u>Directions</u>

1. Add oils to shampoo.

2. Shake thoroughly and use.

ESSENTIAL OIL FOR DOGS' EARS

Doggie Ear Mites

<u>What You Need</u>

1 drop purifying essential oil

1 drop peppermint essential oil

Cotton ball

<u>Directions</u>

1. Apply oils to cotton ball

2. Swab just the inner ear.

Lavender Wax Cleanser

You need to clean dog ears regularly, at least once in a month. This is because Dog ear wax can lead to other ear problems. Besides, it smells terrible and if your dog is outside all day, the dirt can accumulates quickly.

<u>What You Need</u>

5 drops lavender

1 tsp pure witch hazel or vegetable oil

<u>Directions</u>

1. Combine ingredients in a dark bottle.

2. Place several drops on a cotton swab.

3. Remove the surface dirt and then gently remove the wax.

4. Do not stick swab down the ear canal.

5. The mixture can be used for 2-3 cleanings

<u>Wax In The Ear Canal</u>

What do you do when the wax accumulates is the ear canal?

1. Apply 4 drops of the oil mixture above into the ear canal

2. Massage the exterior area of the ear.

3. Your dog will start to shake vigorously but do not worry about this as it will help to bring up the ear wax to the surface where it can easily be cleaned out.

4. Hold your nose! The wax will smell really bad. With regular cleaning however, there will be no need to do this often.

Dog Ear Infection

<u>What You Need</u>

5 drops Melaleuca

5 drops Lavender

5 drops Geranium

1 tbsp coconut oil

<u>Directions</u>

1. Combine all ingredients

2. Clean the ear with a natural cleaner and then use a Q-tip to carefully rub mixture in the ear.

3. Do this two times daily until the infection clears up.

Power Ear Infection Blend
For dogs with long ears

<u>What You Need</u>

4 drops lavender essential oil

7 drops bergamot essential oil

3 drops roman chamomile essential oil

2 drops niaouli or tea tree essential oil

1/2 oz. (15 ml) carrier oil

<u>Directions</u>

1. Combine oils in a dark glass bottle.

2. Drop 2-3 drops into dog's ear canal with a dropper. Massage outside of the ear gently and then use a cotton ball to clean the ear.

3. The dirt in the ear should loosen and wash out. This reduces the risk of ear infections.

SKIN AND COAT ISSUES

Dog Burns
<u>What You Need</u>

3-5 drops Lavender Essential Oil

<u>Directions</u>

1. Make a cold water compress to cool the burn.

2. Apply the oil as soon as possible.

Deodorizing Spray

Use on your dogs if he stinks from prolong outside play. The result is a wonderful smell that will stay with him for days.

<u>What You Need</u>

5 drops Lavender Essential Oil

15 drops Purification Essential Oil

Pinch of Salt

5 oz Water

<u>Directions</u>

1. Add the essential oils to the salt, stirring gently. Now add the water.

2. Spray your dog lightly.

3. This recipe is for dogs weighing over 60 pounds. For smaller dogs, double the amount of carrier oils for a larger dilution ratio.

Dog Abscess

<u>What You Need</u>

2 drops Melaleuca essential oil

2 drops Lavender essential oil

<u>Directions</u>

1. Clean the wound area.

2. Apply Melaleuca essential oil directly on the abscess. Apply several times in a day.

3. Once pus is gone, apply the lavender oil to speed up healing.

Rich Fragrant Shampoo
For dry skin & fleas

<u>What You Need</u>

3 drops peppermint essential oil

2 drops roman chamomile

3 drops lavender essential oil

2 drops Purification

1 drops cedar wood

1 tablespoons castile soap

¼ tsp vitamin E

1 cup water

2 drops citronella (optional, for fleas)

<u>Directions</u>

1. Combine all ingredients in a glass jar. Mixture will be watery with little suds.

2. However, it is gentle and works perfectly. Your dog will smell great for days!

3. To make this a flea and tick shampoo, just add 2drops of citronella essential oil to it.

4. This recipe is for dogs weighing over 60 pounds. For smaller dogs, double the amount of water for a larger dilution ratio.

Wound Blend
For minor cuts, bruises, scrapes and insect bites

<u>What You Need</u>

1 drop Helichrysum

4 drops Lavender

2 drops Niaouli

3 drops sweet marjoram

1/2 oz. (15 ml) olive oil or jojoba oil

<u>Directions</u>

1. Combine and store in a dark glass bottle.

2. Use as needed.

Dog Growths

1. Apply 1 drop Frankincense directly on the growth.

2. Apply undiluted 2 times daily.

Doggie Anti-Itch Blend

To alleviate itching and reduce redness

<u>What You Need</u>

5 drops Lavender essential oil

5 drops Roman Chamomile

2-3 drops Frankincense (optional)

5 oz olive or jojoba oil

3 drops of vitamin E

<u>Directions</u>

1. Combine in a glass dropper bottle.

2. To help soothe the skin, apply 2- to 4 drops to the spot two times daily. For itching apply as needed.

3. This recipe is for dogs weighing over 60 pounds. For smaller dogs, double the amount of carrier oils in the recipe.

Insect Bite Blend

<u>What You Need</u>

10 drops lavender essential oil

2 drops thyme essential oil

4 drops eucalyptus radiata

3 drops German chamomile essential oil

20 drops V-6 vegetable oil complex

<u>Directions:</u>

1. Combine all ingredients in dark glass bottle, turning gently to mix.

2. Apply 1 or 2 drops 2 to 4 times a day for relief.

3. This recipe has only been tested on dogs between 35-55 pounds. Adjust recipe for dogs below 20 pounds or above 60 pounds.

Itchy Skin Remedy

<u>What You Need</u>

7 drops lavender essential oil

2 drops German chamomile essential oil

3 drops geranium essential oil

3 drops carrot seed

Directions:

1. Combine oils and add to 8 oz. (240 ml) of an all-natural shampoo

2. Alternatively add blend to or to 1/2 oz. of any carrier oil.

3. Apply topically on dog's affected skin areas.

Bad Odor Remedy
Keep your dog will smelling fresh and lovely all day long!

What You Need

2 drops Chamomile Roman essential oil

2 drops Geranium essential oil

7-8 drops Lavender essential oil

3 drops Sweet Marjoram essential oil

To 8 oz. (240 ml) all-natural shampoo

Directions:

Combine oils in the shampoo

Power Odor Spray

This quick-and-easy spray will get rid of that nasty dog smell fast!

<u>Directions:</u>

10 drops lavender essential oil

3 drops eucalyptus essential oil

6 drops peppermint essential oil

6 drops sweet orange essential oil

1 cup distilled water

<u>Directions:</u>

1. Add oils to water

2. Mix thoroughly in a spray bottle.

FLEAS AND TICKS

Natural Tick Spritzer

<u>What You Need</u>

1 cup distilled water

2 drops palo santo essential oil

4 drops grapefruit essential oil

2 drops geranium essential oil

1 drop myrrh essential oil

1 drop peppermint essential oil

1 drop castile soap (emollient)

<u>Directions</u>

1. Combine all in a spray bottle, shaking well. Spritz as needed.

2. It is suitable for horses too.

Oregano Tick Removal

1. Apply 1drop of oregano essential oil directly on the tick.

2. The tick should release its grip.

3. If the area is unreachable, place the oil on a cotton swab and then swab the tick.

Flea Control
<u>What You Need</u>

3 drops lemongrass essential oil

3 drops lavender essential oil

3 drops eucalyptus globulus

3 drops lemon essential oil

4 ounces distilled water

4-ounce dark glass spray bottle

Directions

1. Combine all ingredients in a spray bottle, shaking well.

2. Spray on dogs between 35-55 pounds. Adjust recipe for dogs under 20 or over 60 pounds.

3. Rub on areas in the home where fleas usually congregate.

Tick Repellent
What You Need

3 drops bay Leaf essential oil

5 drops geranium essential oil

7 drops lavender essential oil

1/2 oz. (15 ml) sweet almond oil

Directions

Combine and apply 2-3 drops to the tail, neck, chest, back, and legs of your dog.

Calming Mist Spray
Use this recipe to freshen up your dog's coat and remove odors after a long playing day outside.

<u>What You Need</u>

5-10 drops lavender

5-10 drops roman chamomile

10 oz water

<u>Directions</u>

1. Combine in a glass spray bottle.

2. Shake well before application.

Flea and Deodorizing Collar for Dogs
Instant flea and allergy collar!

<u>What You Need</u>

2 drops lavender essential oil

2 drops citronella essential oil

2 drops peppermint essential oil

2 drops purification essential oil

⅓cup purified water

<u>Directions</u>

1. Combine all in a small bowl and soak dog's collar in it.

2. Try not to submerge any plastic pieces as essential oils can degrade plastic.

3. Leave collar to dry and then put it on dog!

4. Store the remaining liquid in a mason jar for use every two weeks.

5. This recipe is for dogs weighing over 60 pounds. For smaller dogs, double the amount of water in the recipe for a larger dilution ratio.

Anti Fleas Shampoo
What You Need

Any doggy shampoo of choice

1-2 drops of lemongrass essential oil

Directions

1. Add the oil to the shampoo and use on pet.

2. You can also add a few drops of the oil to your dog's beddings and blankets when washing or rinsing.

Mosquito Repellent
Mosquitoes transmit heartworm disease in dogs so protect your dogs from them with this homemade repellent.

What You Need

10 drops Myrrh essential oil

20 drops Citronella essential oil

10 drops Rose Geranium essential oil

10 drops Lemongrass essential oil

8 ounces Aloe Vera juice

<u>Directions</u>

1. Combine all in a sprintzer and sprintz on dog's coat daily.

2. be careful to avoid the eye area.

ESSENTIAL OILS FOR EMOTIONS

Like humans, dogs have emotions which are very real to them. Use essential oils to address such emotions like dog anxiety, separation anxiety, fear and stress. They can also be used to calm dogs during thunderstorms and to enliven them during times of loss, depression or separation.

For Calming Dogs
<u>What You Need</u>

1 drop Lavender or Roman Chamomile essential oil

1 drop carrier oil

<u>Directions</u>

1. Mix and rub on dog pads, ears whenever you perceive your dog is stressed.

2. You can also comb through fur.

For Hyperactive Dogs
<u>What You Need</u>

2 drops roman Chamomile essential oil

5 drops lavender essential oil

2 drops bergamot essential oil

3 drops Sweet Marjoram essential oil

3 drops Valerian essential oil

1/2 oz. (15 ml) almond oil or olive oil

<u>Directions</u>

1. Combine all ingredients and then rub 2 to 3 drops between your hands.

2. Apply to dog's inner thighs, the edge of his ears or between the toes.

For Girl Crazy Dogs
Help your dog stay calm and focus with this recipe.

2-3 drops marjoram essential oil

Rub gently on fur

Anxiety Oil Blend

To calm dogs who are afraid of new places, people or things as well as those who suffer from separation anxiety (when an otherwise gentle dog becomes overwrought and destructive when you are not at home) and noise anxiety.

<u>What You Need</u>

2 drops clary sage essential oil

3 drops sweet marjoram essential oil

5 drops lavender essential oil

3 drops valerian essential oil

1/2 oz. (15 ml) jojoba oil, olive oil or sweet almond oil

<u>Directions</u>

1. Combine all ingredients and then rub 2 to 3 drops between your hands.

2. Apply to dog's inner thighs, the edge of his ears or between the toes.

Calming Powder Blend

For stressed dogs and those with anxiety issues.

<u>What You Need</u>

3 parts lavender essential oil

2 parts Melissa essential oil

2 parts bergamot essential oil

1 part ylang ylang essential oil

Baking soda, cornstarch or rice flour

Directions

1. Combine the essential oils. Use 12 to 15 drops of the blend per cup of baking soda.

2. Alternatively, mix baking soda and rice flour together and use per cup for12 to 15 drops essential oil blend flour.

3. Shake or stir to mix well.

How To Use

If your dog is stressed during a car ride, sprinkle the lavender powder blend on a blanket and put it in the cage with the dog.

If your dog suffers from separation anxiety when you are away, sprinkle the powder on any of your old clothes and place it on your dog's bed. Your old clothes emit your smell which reassures your dog while the calming effects of the oil powder blend helps him relax.

For Nervous Exhaustion
Rub 2 to 3 drops lavender essential oil on dog's tummy

ESSENTIAL OILS FOR BONE ISSUES

Joint Pain Relief Blend

1 drop oregano essential oil

5 drops peppermint essential oil

10 drops helichrysum essential oil

30 drops Idaho balsam fir essential oil

<u>Directions</u>

1. Combine all ingredients in dark glass bottle, shaking gently to mix.

 2. Apply 2 to 3 drops to the affected joint thrice daily for relief.

3. This recipe has only been tested on dogs between 35-55 pounds. Adjust recipes for dogs below 20 pounds or above 60 pounds.

Doggie Aging Ointment

As dogs get older, they suffer from aches and pains. This recipe will be helpful for them.

<u>What You Need</u>

3 tbsp coconut oil

3 drops peppermint essential oil

2 drops balsam fir essential oil

3 drops lavender essential oil

2 drops copaiba essential oil

<u>Directions</u>

Make into an ointment and then to rub to the pad of the foot to absorb quickly into the blood stream.

Arthritis Relief
<u>What You Need</u>

3 drops Valerian essential oil

6 drops Helichrysum essential oil

2 drops Ginger essential oil

4 drops Peppermint essential oil

1/2 oz. (15 ml) olive oil, jojoba oil or sweet almond oil

<u>Directions</u>

1. Combine all and massage on dog's sore joints.

2. Apply 1-2 drops on his inner ear tips too.

ESSENTIAL OILS FOR MISCELLANEOUS USES

Immune Support for Allergens

<u>What You Need</u>

1 drop lavender

1 drop peppermint

1 drop lemon

<u>Directions</u>

1. Combine ingredients in an empty capsule.

2. Put it in dog's food or give him directly to swallow

Dog with Sunburned Nose

1-2 drops lavender essential oil

1tsp carrier oil

<u>Directions</u>

Combine and dab on nose for relief.

Sinus Infections

Use this blend to relieve your dog of nasal congestion caused by sinus infection

<u>What You Need</u>

1/2 oz. (15 ml) jojoba oil

5 drops eucalyptus essential oil

5 drops Myrrh essential oil

5 drops Ravensare essential oil

<u>Directions</u>

Combine in a dark glass bottle.

<u>To Use</u>

• Massage 5-7 drops onto dog's chest and neck or place on a cloth bandanna.

• Alternatively, add several drops to the dog's bedding or...

• Let the dog lay on the bathroom floor when you are about to shower. Drop 6-10 drops of the blend onto the shower floor. The steam and vaporized oil will work together to clear the dog's sinus congestion.

• Alternatively, add the only essential oils and not the carrier oils to a diffuser and diffuse for 5 minutes at a time, several times a day.

For Brain Health Support

<u>What You Need</u>

1 drop Frankincense

1 drop lavender

<u>Directions</u>

Apply the Frankincense on spine and the lavender on paws.

Respiratory Support
<u>What You Need</u>

1 drop lime

1 drop thyme

<u>Directions</u>

Combine and apply to the paws.

Dog With A High Fever
<u>What You Need</u>

2-4 drops peppermint essential oil

1 tsp carrier oil

<u>Directions</u>

1. Combine and sprinkle on dog's body.

2. Wrap cool towel over him

Carsick Dogs/ Colic

Rub 2-3 drops peppermint on the tummy.

Motion Sickness

What You Need

6 drops ginger essential oil

6 to 8 drops peppermint essential oil

1/2 oz. (15 ml) olive oil or jojoba oil

Directions

1. Combine and apply onto dog's belly and the inside tip of ears.

2. Also, add 2-3 drops to a cotton ball and place in front of the air vent in the car. Scent will then circulate in the car.